60 Recipes for Protein Snacks for Weightlifters:

Speed up Muscle Growth without Pills, Creatine Supplements, Or Anabolic Steroids

By

Joseph Correa

Certified Sports Nutritionist

COPYRIGHT

© 2016 Correa Media Group

All rights reserved

Reproduction or translation of any part of this work beyond that permitted by section 107 or 108 of the 1976 United States Copyright Act without the permission of the copyright owner is unlawful.

This publication is designed to provide accurate and authoritative information in regard to the subject matter covered. It is sold with the understanding that neither the author nor the publisher is engaged in rendering medical advice. If medical advice or assistance is needed, consult with a doctor. This book is considered a guide and should not be used in any way detrimental to your health. Consult with a physician before starting this nutritional plan to make sure it's right for you.

ACKNOWLEDGEMENTS

The realization and success of this book could not have been possible without my family.

60 Recipes for Protein Snacks for Weightlifters:

Speed up Muscle Growth without Pills, Creatine Supplements, Or Anabolic Steroids

By

Joseph Correa

Certified Sports Nutritionist

CONTENTS

Copyright

Acknowledgements

About The Author

Introduction

60 Recipes for Protein Snacks for Weightlifters: Speed up Muscle Growth without Pills, Creatine Supplements, Or Anabolic Steroids

Other Great Titles by This Author

ABOUT THE AUTHOR

As a certified sports nutritionist and professional athlete, I firmly believe that proper nutrition will help you reach your goals faster and effectively. My knowledge and experience has helped me live healthier throughout the years and which I have shared with family and friends. The more you know about eating and drinking healthier, the sooner you will want to change your life and eating habits.

Being successful in controlling your weight is important as it will improve all aspects of your life.

Nutrition is a key part in the process of getting in better shape and that's what this book is all about.

INTRODUCTION

60 Recipes for Protein Snacks for Weightlifters will help you increase the amount of protein you consume per day to help increase muscle mass. These meals will help increase muscle in an organized manner by adding large healthy portions of protein to your diet. Being too busy to eat right can sometimes become a problem and that's why this book will save you time and help nourish your body to achieve the goals you want. Make sure you know what you're eating by preparing it yourself or having someone prepare it for you.

This book will help you to:

-Gain muscle fast naturally.

-Improve muscle recovery.

-Eat delicious protein snacks.

-Have more energy.

-Naturally accelerate Your Metabolism to build more muscle.

-Improve your digestive system.

Joseph Correa is a certified sports nutritionist and a professional athlete.

60 RECIPES FOR PROTEIN SNACKS FOR WEIGHTLIFTERS

1. Yogurt Pie Delight

Preparing time: 20 minutes
Baking time: 30 minutes
Servings: 15

1. Ingredients:

- **Dough**

500g cottage cheese
6 tablespoon of oats (90g)
4 eggs
2 tablespoon sweetener/honey/brown sugar (30g)
35g yeast
1 tablespoon flour (15g)
200g Greek yogurt
1 tablespoon essence of vanilla/lemon (depending on taste)

- **Stuffing**

3 eggs
2 tablespoon flour (30g)
400g yogurt
2 tablespoon sweetener/honey/brown sugar (30g)
100g raisins

2. Preparation:

In a bowl mix the cottage cheese with the eggs yolk, oats, sweetener (honey/brown sugar), flour, yeast, essence and yogurt. Mix till the composition has a smooth texture.

For the stuffing the eggs whites are mixt till they make foam. Slowly the yolk is added, sweetener (honey/brown sugar), flour, yogurt and raisins.

Prepare the oven at 160 degrees (medium-low level).

Add a baking sheet in a tray and pour half the dough in. Put it in the oven for about 10minutes. When the color of the dough begins to change, remove the tray from the oven and add the stuffing and add it in the oven for another 10min. Finally remove one last time the tray from the oven and add the remaining dough and cook it for another 10min.

3. Nutritional facts (amount per 100g):

Contains Vitamin A, D, C, B-12, B-6, iron, calcium and magnesium.
Calories: 129
  Calories from Fat: 32
Total Fat: 3.6g
  Saturated Fat: 1.5g
Cholesterol: 81mg
Sodium: 189mg
Potassium: 246mg

Total Carbohydrates: 17.2g
    Sugar: 6.7g
Protein: 11.5g

2. Protein marshmallow Punch

Preparing time: 10 minutes
Baking time: 15 minutes
Servings: 5

1. Ingredients:

3 eggs whites
6 tablespoon sweetener (honey/brown sugar) (90g)
50g whey protein
Essence of vanilla/lemon/orange

2. Preparation

The oven is set for 180 degrees Cesium.

Mix the eggs whites till they form a soft foam, then add the sweetener (honey/brown sugar), whey protein and the essence and continue mixing till the composition is hard.

Add the composition in the baking tray with a syringe for decorating cakes, and cook it for about 15 minutes.

3. Nutritional facts (amount per 50g):

Contains Vitamin B-12, iron and magnesium.
Calories: 48
    Calories from Fat: 6
Total Fat: 0.6g

Cholesterol: 21mg
Sodium: 38mg
Potassium: 89mg
Total Carbohydrates: 22.5g
Protein: 9.3g

3. Black waffles with pumpkin

Preparing time: 10 minutes
Baking time: 20 minutes
Servings: 5

1. Ingredients:

2 eggs
1 tablespoon flour (15g)
Sweetener (honey/brown sugar) per taste
2 tablespoon oats (30g)
2 tablespoon cocoa (30g)
2 tablespoon yogurt (30g)
200g mashed pumpkin

2. Preparation:

Add the eggs in a bowl with the sweetener (honey/brown sugar), and mix. Then add the flour and wait for 10minutes till the composition thickens. Then add the rest of the ingredients and mix till all the composition is compact.

Grease the waffle machine and add the composition with a spoon.

3. Nutritional facts (amount per 30g):

Contains Vitamin A, C, D, B-12, B-6, iron, calcium and magnesium.

Fill the muffin forms, about ¾ of the form, but leave some composition behind and mix it with the coffee. This will come on top of the muffin.

Add the muffins in the oven for 35-40 minutes.

3. Nutritional facts (amount per 50g):

Contains: Vitamin A, calcium, iron
Calories: 86
    Calories from Fat: 43
Total Fat: 4.7g
    Saturated Fat: 1.2g
Cholesterol: 39mg
Sodium: 146mg
Potassium: 244mg
Total Carbohydrates: 6.8g
Protein: 7.3g

5. Oats muffins

Preparing time: 10 minutes
Baking time: 15 minutes
Servings: 5

1. Ingredients:

6 tablespoon oats (90g)

2 eggs

100g Greek yogurt

1 tablespoon baking powder (15g)

2 tablespoons cocoa (30g)

4 tablespoons sweetener (honey/brown sugar) (60g)

2. Preparation:

Add the eggs in a bowl and mix them with the yogurt till they smoothen then add the rest of the ingredients and mix them for 5 minutes.

Set the oven beforehand at 180 degree Celsius. The composition is split equal in muffin forms.

Leave them in the oven for about 15 minutes.

3. Nutritional facts (amount per 50g):

Contains Vitamin A, calcium, iron
Calories: 59
    Calories from Fat: 21

Total Fat: 2.4g
    Saturated Fat: 0.9g
Cholesterol: 55mg
Sodium: 29mg
Potassium: 359mg
Total Carbohydrates: 18.2g
    Sugar: 0.9g
Protein: 4.5g

6. Homemade protein bar

Preparing time: 10 minutes
Baking time: 45 minutes
Servings: 5

1. Ingredients:

6-8 tablespoons of whey protein (chocolate/vanilla/ banana) (90-120g)
1 cup oats (240g)
1/3 cup peanut butter (60g)
3 tablespoons honey (45g)
½ cup milk (120g)
3 tablespoons mash almonds (45g)

2. Preparation:

In a bowl mix the whey protein with the oats, peanut butter, honey and milk.

Put the composition in a square tray and stretched it equally. Add the almonds over it.

Put it in the frigid for about 45minutes.

3. Nutritional facts (amount per 100g):

Contains calcium, iron
Calories: 358
    Calories from Fat: 145

Total Fat: 16.1g
   Saturated Fat: 3.4g
Cholesterol: 52mg
Sodium: 135mg
Potassium: 393mg
Total Carbohydrates: 30.8g
   Sugar: 14.3g
Protein: 26.3g

7. Oat Cookies

Preparing time: 10 minutes
Baking time: 35 minutes
Servings: 20

1. Ingredients:

140g butter (80% fat)

50g sugar

70g brown sugar

1 tablespoon honey (15g)

1 tablespoon milk (15g)

140g flour

2g sodium bicarbonate

1 tablespoon baking powder (15g)

100g oats

30g whey protein

1 tablespoon chocolate 70% cacao (mash) (15g)

1 tablespoon ginger/cinnamon/nutmeg (15g)

2. Preparation:

Set the oven at 160degree Celsius.

In a bowl mix the butter with the white and brown sugar, and mix for 2-3minutes. Add the honey and milk and mix. Add the chocolate.

The flour is mixt with the baking powder, whey protein and sodium bicarbonate and then added over the butter.

Add the ginger/cinnamon/nutmeg and mix slow.

You will obtain a dough and on it add the oats, and mix till there are incorporated.

With your hands make small balls (smaller then a ping-pong ball) and put them on the tray (before put a baking sheet in).

Let the cookies bake for 25-30 minutes at 160degree Celsius.

3. Nutritional facts (amount per 50g):

Contains Vitamin A, calcium, iron
Calories: 232
    Calories from Fat: 101
Total Fat: 11.2g
    Saturated Fat: 6.8g
Cholesterol: 33mg
Sodium: 83mg
Potassium: 213mg
Total Carbohydrates: 29.3g
    Sugar: 12.6g
Protein: 4.7g

8. Dried Apricot Cookies

Preparing time: 10 minutes
Baking time: 15 minutes
Servings: 40

1. Ingredients:

120g butter
200g brown sugar
1 tablespoon baking powder (15g)
½ tablespoon cinnamon (7g)
1 egg
1 teaspoon vanilla essence (5g)
2 tablespoon honey (30g)
135g whole wheat flour
90g oats
60g dried apricot (mash)
90g whey protein

2. *Preparation:*

In a bowl mix the butter with 150g brown sugar. Mix until the composition has a creamy aspect.

Add the vanilla essence, egg and honey. Mix for 2-3 minutes and then add the two types of flower, baking powder, whey protein and dried apricot.

Mix until the composition smoothens.

The dough is move in a new bowl and it's covered with a food foil and left in the fridge for at least 1h, it can also be left overnight.

After the time is finish, form small balls (nuts size). The resulting balls are roll in the remaining 50g brown sugar.

Cover two trays with baking sheets and add the ball on it. Put the balls at a 5-6cm distances between them.

Put the trays in the preheated oven at 180degree Celsius.

3. *Nutritional facts (amount per 20g):*

Contains Vitamin A, C, calcium and iron
Calories: 76
    Calories from Fat: 26
Total Fat: 2.9g
    Saturated Fat: 1.7g
Cholesterol: 15mg
Sodium: 25mg
Potassium: 77mg
Total Carbohydrates: 10.6g
    Sugar: 6g
Protein: 2.5g

9. Almond cookies

Preparing time: 1:30 hour
Baking time: 30 minutes

1. Ingredients:
180g almonds
250g whole wheat flour
125g butter
200g brown sugar
3 eggs
2 tablespoons baking powder (30g)
3-4 drops of almond extract

2. Preparation:

First you need to add the almonds in a preheated oven at 180 degrees Celsius for about 5minutes. Remove them from the oven and let the cool off for 5minutes and before you add the in the food processor you need to rub them between your palms and you'll see that the skin will come off.

After you mix the almonds in the food processor you add the brown sugar, flour, baking powder and mix again for a couple of minutes.

When the composition in the robot looks like it compact you add the eggs and the almond essence.

The result will be a sticky dough.

You will break the composition in half and put it in a food foil. Wrap the foil in a cylindrical shape with a 4cm diameter.

The result foil will go in the fridge for 1houre.

After 1houre has pass heat the oven at 175degrees Celsius.

Remove one cylinder at a time from the fridge. Clear the food foil from it and cut it in pieces of 7-8mm thick. Put them on a tray cover with baking paper.

Add them in the oven for about 15minutes, then flip them and leave them for another 10-15 minutes in the oven.

Repeat the process for the second dough.

3. Nutritional facts (amount per 100g):

Contains Vitamin A, calcium, Iron
Calories: 425
    Calories from Fat: 207
Total Fat: 23g
    Saturated Fat: 8.4g
Cholesterol: 84mg
Sodium: 111mg
Potassium: 565mg
Total Carbohydrates: 49g
    Sugar: 22.6g

Protein: 9.1g

10. Avocado Truffles

Preparing time: 30 minutes

1. Ingredients:
200g chocolate (70% cocoa)
3-4 tablespoon cocoa powder (45-60g)
50g almond (crushed)
½ cup avocado (mesh)(120g)
½ tablespoon vanilla essence (7g)
5g salt

2. Preparation:

The dark chocolate is melted a bain-marie (water bath). Add the vanilla extract and the salt and waist till the chocolate is smooth.

Mesh the avocado and mix it with the melted chocolate until the composition has thickened.

Place the result in the fridge for about 20 minutes.

Use a tablespoon to remove the composition from the bowl and give them a ball shape. Roll them in the cocoa powder or almond. Store them in the fridge and serve them at room temperature.

3. Nutritional facts (amount per 50g):

Contains : Vitamin A, C, iron, calcium
Calories: 223
    Calories from Fat: 129
Total Fat: 14.4g
    Saturated Fat: 6.8g
Cholesterol: 7mg
Sodium: 299mg
Potassium: 269mg
Total Carbohydrates: 20.8g
    Sugar: 15.2g
Protein: 4.3g

11. Almond and Orange Cookies

Preparing time: 20 minutes
Baking time: 40 minutes

1. Ingredients:

100g almonds

50g butter

115g brown sugar

1 egg

15ml orange juice

Rind from 1 small orange

175g oats

1 tablespoon baking powder (10g)

40g polenta

2. Preparation:

Preheat the oven at 170 degrees Celsius. On a baking sheet put the almonds and bake them for 10-15 minutes (until golden). Cool them for 5 minutes and the chop them in small pieces.

The butter is mixed with the sugar.

In a separate bowl mix the egg with the juice and the orange rind. Mix them with the butter.

Add the oats, baking powder, milk and polenta and mix until the dough has a soft texture.

Place the dough on a baking sheet and sprinkle with the chop almonds. Place it in the oven for about 30minutes.

Cut the cookies and place them for another 10minutes in the oven until crisp.

3. Nutritional facts (amount per 50g):
Contains calcium, iron, Vitamin A
Calories: 206
    Calories from Fat: 87
Total Fat: 9.7g
    Saturated Fat: 3g
Cholesterol: 25mg
Sodium: 37mg
Potassium: 282mg
Total Carbohydrates: 26.6g
    Sugar: 10.8g
Protein: 4.8g

12. Banana muffins

Preparing time: 10 minutes
Baking time: 15 minutes
Servings: 16

1. Ingredients:
2 banana
500g cottage cheese
2 eggs

2. Preparation:

Mix all the ingredients in a bowl till you obtain a smooth composition. Pour the composition in the muffin forms and add them in the preheated oven at 190 degrees Celsius for 15 minutes (till the side is color in a light brown shade).

3. Nutritional facts (amount per 50g):
Contains : Vitamin A, C, iron, calcium
Calories: 49
    Calories from Fat: 11
Total Fat: 1.2g
    Saturated Fat: 0.6g
Cholesterol: 23mg
Sodium: 135mg
Potassium: 90mg
Total Carbohydrates: 4.5g

Sugar: 1.9g
Protein: 5.1g

13. Peanut Butter and Banana Pudding

Preparing time: 10 minutes
Waiting time: 4 hours
Servings: 3

1. Ingredients:

500ml milk

15g corn starch

50g sweetener (honey/brown sugar)

10g peanut butter

2 tablespoons lemon juice (30g)

250g banana

50g whey protein

4 gelatin sheets

2. Preparation:

Soak the gelatin sheets in cold water.

Put some water to boil in a pan. In a deferent bowl mix the milk, corn starch, whey protein, sweetener (honey/brown sugar) and peanut butter.

Add the bowl on the pan with the boil water and mix till you obtain a cream. The bowl doesn't have to touch the water surface.

Remove the bowl from the pan and add the gelatin sheets and mix for 1minut. Add a food foil directly on the composition and leave it to cool down.

Slice the bananas and pour over them the lemon juice.

Distribute some (about 3 tablespoon) composition in 3 glasses and add the bananas over the composition (75g in each glass). Then divide the rest of the composition into the 3 glasses and sprinkle some peanut over them.

Put the glasses in the fridge and let them cool for at least 4hours.

3. Nutritional facts (amount per 100g):
Contains Vitamin C, iron, calcium
Calories: 90
    Calories from Fat: 20
Total Fat: 2.2g
    Saturated Fat: 1.1g
Cholesterol: 16mg
Sodium: 44mg
Potassium: 175mg
Total Carbohydrates: 18.2g
    Sugar: 6.3g
Protein: 6.8g

14. Banana and Dried Apricot Pancakes

Preparing time: 5 minutes
Baking time: 5 minutes
Servings: 1

1. Ingredients:

- Pancake

160g banana
2 eggs
15g sweetener (honey/brown sugar)
50g whey protein

- Yogurt cream

150g Greek yogurt
100g dried apricot
10g sweetener (honey/brown sugar)

- Topping

20g almonds

2. Preparation:

Separate the egg whites from yolks.

Mix the yolks with bananas, whey protein and sweetener (honey/brown sugar), until the composition becomes creamy.

The eggs whites are mix until they are foam and then we add them onto the yolks, mixing slowly.

On a silicon tray place the composition in 2-3 pancakes shapes and add them in the microwave oven for about 5minutes.

Mix the Greek yogurt with sweetener (honey/brown sugar) and apricot. Place it on the pancakes; spay some nuts or maple syrup on top.

3. Nutritional facts (amount per 100g):
Contains Vitamin A, C, calcium, iron
Calories: 104
    Calories from Fat: 24
Total Fat: 2.7g
    Saturated Fat: 1.1g
Cholesterol: 73mg
Sodium: 44mg
Potassium: 241mg
Total Carbohydrates: 14.9g
    Sugar: 6.1g
Protein: 10.8g

15. Protein pancakes

Preparing time: 5 minutes
Baking time: 10 minutes
Servings: 1

1. Ingredients:

45g oat flour

25g coconut flour

1 tablespoon baking powder (15g)

30g sweetener (honey/brown sugar)

120g cottage cheese

4 egg whites

1 tablespoon banana essence (15g)

½ tablespoon vanilla powder (7g)

10 g caramel syrup

Pinch of salt

2. Preparation:

Mix the oats flour with the coconut flour, sweetener (honey/brown sugar), salt and baking powder.

Add the cottage cheese, eggs whites, banana essence, vanilla powder and mix for 2-3 minutes.

Whit a tablespoon add composition in a pan grease with butter or oil.

Let the pancake cook on each side for 1-2minutes.

Use bananas, maple syrup, honey of fruits as topping.

3. Nutritional facts (amount per 100g):
Contains calcium, iron;
Calories: 123
    Calories from Fat: 19
Total Fat: 2.1g
    Saturated Fat: 1g
Cholesterol: 2mg
Sodium: 198mg
Potassium: 501mg
Total Carbohydrates: 25g
    Sugar: 1g
Protein: 10.1g

16. Half Baked Banana Cheesecake

Preparing time: 15 minutes
Baking time: 15 minutes
Waiting time: 4 hours
Servings: 8

1. Ingredients:

- Dough

100g oats

10g cacao powder

3 eggs

1 tablespoon milk (15g)

1 teaspoon baking powder (15g)

1 tablespoon sweetener (honey/brown sugar) (15g)

- Cream

250g cottage cheese

400g Greek yogurt

300g bananas

2 tablespoons sweetener (honey/brown sugar) (30g)

12 gelatin sheets

½ teaspoon vanilla powder (2.5g)

2. Preparation:

For the dough mix all the ingredients, and put the composition in a round tray and cook it in a preheated oven at 180degree Celsius for 15minutes.

The gelatin will be put in cold water.

For the cream add all the ingredients in a bowl and mix till you obtain a smooth cream.

Remove the water from the gelatin and put it in the microwave for 10-15 minutes.

Add the gelatin in to the cream and mix very well.

Put the cream over the cook dough and add the result in the fridge for 4hours.

3. Nutritional facts (amount per 100g):
Contains Vitamin A, C, calcium, iron
Calories: 120
　　Calories from Fat: 27
Total Fat: 3g
　　Saturated Fat: 1.3g
Cholesterol: 44mg
Sodium: 114mg
Potassium: 245mg
Total Carbohydrates: 18.6g
　　Sugar: 4.7g
Protein: 10g

17. Banana and peanuts cake

Preparing time: 15 minutes
Baking time: 40-50 minutes

1. Ingredients:
300g peanut flour
310g banana puree
120g apple puree
5 eggs
85g peanut butter
80g coconut milk
100g sweetener (honey/brown sugar)
10g baking powder

2. Preparation:

In a bowl mix the almond flour with the baking powder and sweetener (honey/brown sugar).

Mesh the bananas and the peanut butter, coconut milk, eggs and mix till smoothen.

Add the bananas on the flour and mix for 2 minutes.

Pour the composition in a round tray and cook it for 40-50 minutes at 180degree Celsius.

3. Nutritional facts (amount per 100g):
Contains Vitamin A, calcium, iron

Calories: 235
    Calories from Fat: 124
Total Fat: 13.8g
    Saturated Fat: 3.5g
Cholesterol: 68mg
Sodium: 78mg
Potassium: 511mg
Total Carbohydrates: 21g
    Sugar: 11.5g
Protein: 12.7g

18. Apple and oats cake

Preparing time: 25 minutes
Baking time: 45-50 minutes
Servings: 8

1. Ingredients:

120g oat
100g brown rice flour
50g oats flakes
120g apple puree
5 eggs whites
200g milk
2 tablespoon sweetener (honey/brown sugar) (30g)
1 teaspoon vanilla essence (5g)
10g baking powder
½ teaspoon cinnamon (2.5g)
240g apple

2. Preparation:

In a bowl add the oats, rice flour and baking powder and mix. Add the apple puree, egg whites, milk, sweetener (honey/brown sugar), vanilla essence and cinnamon and mix for another 2 minutes.

Put the composition in a round tray and sprinkle the oats flakes on it. The apple will be cut in a crescent form about 2-3mm thick and place on top of the cake.

Cook the cake for 45-50 minutes in a preheated oven at 180 degree Celsius.

3. *Nutritional facts (amount per 100g):*
Contains : Vitamin C, calcium, iron
Calories: 139
   Calories from Fat: 17
Total Fat: 1.9g
   Saturated Fat: 0.5g
Cholesterol: 2mg
Sodium: 29mg
Potassium: 255mg
Total Carbohydrates: 27.4g
   Sugar: 5g
Protein: 5.5g

19. Brownies

Preparing time: 60 minutes
Baking time: 10 minutes
Servings: 6

1. Ingredients:

120g oats flour
80g chocolate (melted)
186g apple puree
120g brown sugar
3 eggs
5g baking powder

2. Preparation:

All the ingredients are added in a bowl and mix for 4-6 minutes.

Pour the composition in a tray and add it in an oven preheated at 180degree Celsius for 50minutes.

You can serve them cool or warm, they very good either way.

3. Nutritional facts (amount per 100g):
Contains Vitamin C, calcium, iron
Calories: 275
   Calories from Fat: 68
Total Fat: 7.5g

    Saturated Fat: 3.8g
Cholesterol: 85mg
Sodium: 48mg
Potassium: 260mg
Total Carbohydrates: 45.8g
    Sugar: 29.7g
Protein: 6.6g

20. Mini Cheesecakes

Preparing time: 15 minutes
Waiting time: 4 hours
Servings: 5

1. Ingredients:

- **Strawberry jelly**

150g strawberry

30g sweetener (honey/brown sugar)

3 gelatin sheets

- **Yogurt cream**

100g Greek yogurt

2 gelatin sheets

30g sweetener (honey/brown sugar)

30g strawberries

- **Dough**

57g digestive biscuit

2 tablespoon of strawberry jelly (30g)

2. Preparation:

A. Jelly

Put all the gelatin sheets in water.

Put all the strawberry (cut in small pieces) in a pan. Add the sweetener (honey/brown sugar) and put them on the stove. Stir continues for 2-3 minutes.

With the help of a mixer transform the composition a puree, and add 3 gelatin sheets, and mix till the gelatin is dissolve.

B. Dough

Smash the biscuits (in a blander) and add 2 teaspoons of jelly (the one that you just finish making). And mix till the composition is smooth.

Split the composition in 3 equal pieces (in square or round forms) and press the dough very well.

C. Yogurt Cream

Mix the yogurt with the sweetener (honey/brown sugar) till it's completely dissolves.

Melt the gelatin in the microwave; put a tablespoon of yogurt in it, to lower its temperature and be easier to mix.

Add the strawberry's cut in small pieces and mix all the ingredients till the composition is creamy.

D. Assembly

Put equal yogurt cream on the 3 pieces of dough. Put the cake in the fridge for 40minutes.

Add the jelly, and put the cake into the fridge, till the jelly hardens. It will take about 3 hours.

3. Nutritional facts (amount per 100g):
Contains Vitamin A, C, calcium, iron;
Calories: 134
    Calories from Fat: 29
Total Fat: 3.2g
    Saturated Fat: 0.8g
Cholesterol: 4mg
Sodium: 82mg
Potassium: 94mg
Total Carbohydrates: 29.7g
    Sugar: 10.2g
Protein: 11.5g

21. Cacao and almonds desert

Preparing time: 30 minutes
Cooking time: 30 minutes
Servings: 8

1. Ingredients:

- Dough

136g flour
120g black rice flour
40g corn starch
10g baking powder
2 teaspoon cinnamon (30g)
260g pumpkin puree
250ml coconut milk
¾ cup egg white (180g)
100g sweetener (honey/brown sugar)
Pinch of salt

- Cream

250g Greek yogurt
200ml coconut milk
25g cacao powder
150g almond flour
10g sweetener (honey/brown sugar)

2. Preparation:

In a bowl add the pumpkin puree, egg white, coconut milk, sweetener (honey/brown sugar), salt and essence and mix for 2-3 minutes.

In a smaller bowl add the flour, rice flour, baking powder, starch and cinnamon and mix till smooth.

Combine the two bowls and mix for 3-4 minutes increasing the mixer speed.

The dough will be put in two trays equally. The trays need to be the same size. And bake them for 30minutes at 180degree Celsius.

For the cream mix all the ingredients till there smooth.

When the dough cools down we began the assembly. First one dough then cream then the next dough and at the end all the remaining cream goes on top and on the side.

Put the cake in the fridge for 30minutes.

3. *Nutritional facts (amount per 100g):*
Contains Vitamin A, C, calcium, iron
Calories: 166
    Calories from Fat: 79
Total Fat: 8.4g
    Saturated Fat: 6.2g
Cholesterol: 1mg
Sodium: 30mg
Potassium: 215mg

Total Carbohydrates: 26.6g
   Sugar: 2.2g
Protein: 5.5g

22. Almond and Chocolate cake

Preparing time: 30 minutes
Cooking time: 40 minutes
Servings: 8

1. Ingredients:

- Dough

6 eggs whites
150g sweetener (honey/brown sugar)
50g oats
40g almond flakes
Pinch of salt

- Cream

100g whey protein (chocolate flavor)
15g cacao powder
20g powdered milk
150g avocado
150g quark
50g sweetener (honey/brown sugar)

- Decoration

10g almond flakes
5g dark chocolate

2. Preparation:

A. Dough

In a bowl mix the egg whites with salt till you have fluffy foam. Add gradually the sweetener (honey/brown sugar) stirring continue. And mix till the foam becomes firm.

Mix the oat flour with almond flakes and add them to the egg whites composition

Split the composition in two equal trays and bake it for 35-40 minutes at 180degree Celsius.

B. Cream

Mix all the ingredients in a blender till smoothen.

C. Assembly

Place the first dough on and add 2/3 of the cream on it. Add the second dough and the rest of the cream on it.

Decorate the sides with almond flakes and grated chocolate.

Let the cake in the fridge for 8hours or even better overnight.

3. Nutritional facts (amount per 100g):
Contains Vitamin C, calcium, iron
Calories: 184
    Calories from Fat: 88
Total Fat: 9.7g
    Saturated Fat: 2.6g
Cholesterol: 28mg

Sodium: 95mg
Potassium: 202mg
Total Carbohydrates: 36.1g
    Sugar: 2.8g
Protein: 15.5g

23. Raspberry desert

Preparing time: 3 minutes
Waiting time: 8 hours
Servings: 1

1. Ingredients:

40g oats
50g whey protein
40g sweetener (honey/brown sugar)
100g raspberries
100g cheese cream
100ml milk
100ml water
½ teaspoon raspberry essence (2.5g)

2. Preparation:

Mix oats with whey protein, sweetener (honey/brown sugar) and raspberry. Add the rest of the ingredients and mix till the composition is smooth.

Cover the bowl with food foil and add it to the fridge for 8hours or overnight.

3. Nutritional facts (amount per 100g):
Contains Vitamin A, C, calcium, iron
Calories: 156
    Calories from Fat: 75
Total Fat: 8.3g
    Saturated Fat: 4.6g

Cholesterol: 43mg
Sodium: 96mg
Potassium: 128mg
Total Carbohydrates: 20.8g
    Sugar: 2.9g
Protein: 10.4g

24. Chocolate mouse

Preparing time: 20 minutes
Waiting time: 3 hours
Servings: 4

1. Ingredients:

4 eggs
250g cottage cheese
60g whey protein (chocolate)
10g cacao powder
100g sweetener (honey/brown sugar)
10 gelatin sheets
2 teaspoons mint essence (30g)
1 teaspoon matcha (15g)
2-3 drops natural food coloring (green)
Pinch of salt

2. Preparation:

Put the gelatin sheets in cold water.

Separate the yolk from the egg whites in two bowls.

Mix the yolks with 50g sweetener (honey/brown sugar) till they double in volume. Add the cottage cheese and mix till smooth.

Place the bowl on top of a pan with boil water (make sure the bowl is heat resistant), mixing continue. The cream is ready when it's thick, it will take about 5 minutes.

Remove the cream from the pan and add the gelatin sheets, and mix till the gelatin is dissolve.

Mix the egg whites till the foam is soft then add the rest of the sweetener (honey/brown sugar) and salt, and mix till the foam is hard.

Add the egg whites foam to the yolk cream.

2/3 of the composition will be used for the chocolate mousse and 1/3 for the mint mousse.

In the 2/3 go the whey protein, cacao, and mix till it's smooth. Put half of the composition in a pastry syringe and fill the glasses with a layer of chocolate mousse. And place the glasses in the freezer for 10minutes.

For the mint mousse we add the mint essence, matcha and coloring. Put all the composition in another pastry syringe and add another layer in every glass. Put the glasses in the freezer for 5-10minutes.

Put the rest of the chocolate mousse in the glasses. Put the mousse in the fridge for 3 hours.

3. Nutritional facts (amount per 100g):
Contains Vitamin A, calcium, iron

Calories: 130
    Calories from Fat: 42
Total Fat: 4.7g
    Saturated Fat: 1.9g
Cholesterol: 133mg
Sodium: 259mg
Potassium: 136mg
Total Carbohydrates: 23.8g
    Sugar: 1g
Protein: 18.3g

25. Coconut and Quinoa Pudding

Preparing time: 3 minutes
Cooking time: 30 minutes
Servings: 4-6

1. Ingredients:

½ cup quinoa (120g)

50g whey protein

½ vanilla bean (scrape)

1/5 cup sugar (25g)

100ml coconut milk

Pinch of salt

2. Preparation:

In a pan add the coconut milk, sugar, whey protein and vanilla.

Cook until the milk comes to simmer. Add the quinoa (rise in cold water). Stir every few minutes for 30minutes on the stove set on low.

The pudding is ready when the quinoa blooms and the milk reduce to a pudding consistency.

3. Nutritional facts (amount per 50g):

Contains Vitamin C, calcium, iron
Calories: 148
    Calories from Fat: 49
Total Fat: 5.4g

    Saturated Fat: 3.9g
Cholesterol: 17mg
Sodium: 45mg
Potassium: 171mg
Total Carbohydrates: 17.7g
    Sugar: 7.5g
Protein: 8.3g

26. Quinoa Brownies

Preparing time: 15 minutes
Cooking time: 40 minutes
Servings: 8-16

1. Ingredients:

2/3 cup quinoa (150g)

1 1/3 cup milk (310g)

1/3 cup almond milk (70g)

3 eggs

1 teaspoon pure vanilla extracts (5g)

200g butter

1 1/2 cup coconut palm sugar (340g)

1 cup cocoa powder (230g)

1 ½ teaspoon baking powder (8g)

½ teaspoon baking soda (3g)

½ teaspoon salt (3g)

2. Preparation:

Preheat the oven at 180degree Celsius.

In a blander combine milk, eggs and vanilla. Add the quinoa and butter and mix until smooth.

In a bowl mix sugar, cocoa, baking powder, baking soda and salt. Add the quinoa cream over and mix well.

Put all the composition on a tray and bake for 40minutes.

3. Nutritional facts (amount per 100g):

Contains Vitamin A, calcium, iron
Calories: 289
    Calories from Fat: 219
Total Fat: 24.4g
    Saturated Fat: 15g
Cholesterol: 105mg
Sodium: 369mg
Potassium: 464mg
Total Carbohydrates: 16.2g
    Sugar: 2.3g
Protein: 6.9g

27. Raspberry cake

Preparing time: 25 minutes
Waiting time: 8 hours
Servings: 8

1. Ingredients:

- Dough

100g nuts

150g dried dates

50g dried persimmon

100g coconut flour

50g sweetener (honey/brown sugar)

60ml milk

- Raspberry jelly

200g raspberry

40g sweetener (honey/brown sugar)

5 sheets gelatin

- Chocolate ganache

50g cocoa powder

60g sweetener (honey/brown sugar)

15g powder milk

120ml milk

30g coconut oil

2. Preparation:

A. Dough

In a blander mix the nuts till they become flour consistence. Add the rest of the ingredients and mix till smooth.

In a round tray place food foil on the bottom and the pour the result composition. Distribute equally on the surface. Put the tray in the fridge.

B. Raspberry jelly

Put the gelatin sheets in cold water.

Mix the raspberry with sweetener (honey/brown sugar) in a pan on a low flame, mixing continue. Smash the raspberry and remove the pan from the oven. Add the gelatin and mix till its dissolve.

Wait till the jelly cools down then add it on to the dough, and put the tray back in the fridge.

C. Ganache

Mix the cacao with sweetener (honey/brown sugar) and powder milk. Add the melted coconut oil.

Put the milk in and mix for 1-2 minutes. You will obtain a creamy composition.

Pour the composition in the tray and put the tray back in the fridge for 8hours.

3. Nutritional facts (amount per 100g):
Contains Vitamin C, A, calcium, iron
Calories: 236
  Calories from Fat: 104
Total Fat: 11.5g
  Saturated Fat: 5.2g
Cholesterol: 2mg
Sodium: 111mg
Potassium: 359mg
Total Carbohydrates: 45.8g
  Sugar: 12.2g
Protein: 10.5g

28. Cherry cupcakes

Preparing time: 5 minutes
Cooking time: 25 minutes
Servings: 8

1. Ingredients:

50g almond flour
50g coconut flour
50g black rice flour
50g sweetener (honey/brown sugar)
15g corn starch
10g baking powder
250ml coconut milk
3 egg whites
100g quark
150g cherries

2. Preparation:

Remove the seeds from the cherries.

Mix all the flours with the corn starch, sweetener (honey/brown sugar) and baking powder.

Add the rest of the ingredient except the cherries, and mix for 2-3 minutes

Put 2 tablespoon in each muffin shape and add the cherries (you can also press them in the composition).

Cook them for 25minutes in a preheated oven at 180degree Celsius.

3. *Nutritional facts (amount per 100g):*
Contains Vitamin A, C, calcium, iron;
Calories: 186
    Calories from Fat: 95
Total Fat: 10.6g
    Saturated Fat: 7.9g
Cholesterol: 3mg
Sodium: 41mg
Potassium: 254mg
Total Carbohydrates: 27g
    Sugar: 1.7g
Protein: 4.9g

29. Strawberry cupcakes

Preparing time: 5 minutes
Cooking time: 25-30 minutes
Servings: 6

1. Ingredients:

100g oats
50g black rice flour
15g corn starch
50g sweetener (honey/brown sugar)
½ teaspoon vanilla (3g)
1 egg
100g apple puree
100ml coconut milk
1 tablespoon strawberry essence (15g)
80g strawberry gem

2. Preparation:

Mix the oats flour with the rice flour, corn starch, sweetener (honey/brown sugar) and vanilla.

Add egg, coconut milk, strawberry essence and apple puree, and mix for 2-3minutes.

Split the composition equally in muffin forms add 1 tablespoon of strawberry gem in each, mixing so that the gem will be incorporated.

Cook the muffins for 25-30minutes in a preheated oven at 180degree Celsius.

3. Nutritional facts (amount per 100g):
Contains Vitamin A, C. calcium, iron
Calories: 195
    Calories from Fat: 65
Total Fat: 7.2g
    Saturated Fat: 4.8g
Cholesterol: 33mg
Sodium: 21mg
Potassium: 146mg
Total Carbohydrates: 40.1g
    Sugar: 4.4g
Protein: 5g

30. Proteins balls

Preparing time: 10 minutes
Waiting time: 4 hours
Servings: 30

1. Ingredients:

400g chickpeas

60g coconut flour

30g whey protein

100g sweetener (honey/brown sugar)

50ml coconut milk

2. Preparation:

The chickpeas go in a blender and you will mix it until it becomes a paste.

Put the paste in a bowl and add the rest of the ingredients. Mix all the composition till smooth. Form a large ball and cover it with food foil, and put the bowl in the fridge for 4hours.

With a teaspoon we take composition from the bowl and form small balls.

3. Nutritional facts (amount per 20g):
Contains Vitamin C, calcium, iron
Calories: 65
    Calories from Fat: 13
Total Fat: 1.5

    Saturated Fat: 0.6g
Cholesterol: 2mg
Sodium: 5mg
Potassium: 127mg
Total Carbohydrates: 13.6g
    Sugar: 1.5g
Protein: 3.6g

31. Raffaello

Preparing time: 15 minutes
Waiting time: 8 hours
Servings: 30

1. Ingredients:

200g cottage cheese

200g Greek yogurt

20g psyllium husk

50g whey protein

100g powder milk

100g sweetener (honey/brown sugar)

20g oats

1 tablespoon coconut essence (15g)

30 almonds

100g coconut flakes

2. Preparation:

In a pan fry the almonds, till the peel goes off.

50g coconut flakes are mix with cottage cheese, whey protein, Greek yogurt, powder milk, sweetener (honey/brown sugar), psyllium husk and coconut essence. Cover the bowl in aluminum foil and put it in the fridge for at least 6hours, or better overnight.

With a teaspoon we take some composition and in the middle an almond and so we form 30 small balls they also go through the remaining coconut flakes.

3. *Nutritional facts (amount per 25g):*
Contains calcium, iron
Calories: 50
    Calories from Fat: 24
Total Fat: 2.6g
    Saturated Fat: 1.1g
Cholesterol: 4mg
Sodium: 38mg
Potassium: 76mg
Total Carbohydrates: 6.7g
    Sugar: 0.5g
Protein: 3.4g

32. Digestive Biscuit

Preparing time: 10 minutes
Cooking time: 15 minutes

1. Ingredients:

220g oats
80g peanut butter
2 egg whites
100ml milk
1 tablespoon sweetener (honey/brown sugar) (15g)
6g almonds

2. Preparation:

Put the oats in a blender and mix them.

Over them add peanut butter, egg whites, milk, and sweetener (honey/brown sugar) and mix well.

Whit a tablespoon take some composition form a ball and then add it on a tray, repeat the process till you have no more composition.

Take half of almond and place it in the middle of the cookie.

Cook the biscuits for 15minutes in a preheated oven at 180degree Celsius.

3. Nutritional facts (amount per 100g):

Contains calcium, iron
Calories: 285
 Calories from Fat: 108
Total Fat: 12g
 Saturated Fat: 2.5g
Cholesterol: 2mg
Sodium: 99mg
Potassium: 305mg
Total Carbohydrates: 37.8g
 Sugar: 3g
Protein: 12.2g

33. Almond, persimmon and raisins bars

Preparing time: 15 minutes
Waiting time: 1 day
Servings: 10

1. Ingredients:

200g persimmon
50g nuts
50g raisins
50g almonds
100g coconut flour
50g oats
20g psyllium husk
200ml milk
50g sweetener (honey/brown sugar)

2. Preparation:

Put the persimmon in a bowl with 300ml milk (warm) and let the rehydrate for 4hours.

After 4 hours remove the persimmon and press them with a towel to remove the milk from them. Add them in a blender with the nuts and raisins. Mix till they become a thick paste.

In a bowl mix the coconut flour with oat flour and psyllium husk, add the milk from the persimmon and mix, add the sweetener (honey/brown sugar), and mix again.

Put the composition in a square form and cover it with food foil. Put it in the fridge and leave it overnight.

The next day cut the composition.

3. *Nutritional facts (amount per 100g):*
Contains Vitamin C, calcium, iron
Calories: 219
    Calories from Fat: 79
Total Fat: 8.7g
    Saturated Fat: 1.9g
Cholesterol: 2mg
Sodium: 61mg
Potassium: 245mg
Total Carbohydrates: 40.3g
    Sugar: 5.5g
Protein: 6.2g

34. Oats and cashew bars

Preparing time: 5 minutes
Waiting time: 8 hours
Servings: 14

1. Ingredients:

150g persimmons
200ml milk (warm)
200g oats
100g cashew
30g sweetener (honey/brown sugar)
1 teaspoon vanilla essence (5g)

2. Preparation:

Put the persimmon in 200ml milk and leave them in for 8hours. After 8hourse put them in a blender, and mix till there smooth.

Put the composition in a bowl and add sweetener (honey/brown sugar) and mix. Add the cashew and oats, and mix till smooth.

Put the composition in a tray, cover it with food foil and put it in the fridge for 8 hours, or overnight. After it cool down cut it in pieces.

3. Nutritional facts (amount per 50g):

Contains Vitamin C, a, calcium, iron

Calories: 49
    Calories from Fat: 41
Total Fat: 4.6g
    Saturated Fat: 1g
Cholesterol: 1mg
Sodium: 9mg
Potassium: 134mg
Total Carbohydrates: 18.9g
    Sugar: 1.2g
Protein: 3.5g

35. Cake with lemon flavor

Preparing time: 45 minutes
Cooking time: 15 minutes
Servings: 14

1. Ingredients:

- Dough

150g oats flour

50g rice flour

20g starch

1 teaspoon vanilla powder

1 teaspoon lemon essence

1 egg

2 egg whites

120g apple puree

100ml coconut milk

50g sweetener (honey/brown sugar)

- Cream

300g quark

200g cottage cheese

70g sweetener (honey/brown sugar)

20g psyllium husk

- Syrup

150ml water

10g sweetener (honey/brown sugar)

2. Preparation:

A. Dough

In a bowl mix oat flour, rice flour, starch, vanilla powder and sweetener (honey/brown sugar).

In a small bowl mix all wet ingredients. And then add them on the flour.

Put all the composition in a large tray and put it in a preheated oven at 180degree Celsius for 15-20minutes.

Let it cool down then cut it in 3 equal pieces.

B. Cream

Mix the quark with the cottage cheese, add gradually the psyllium husk and mix for another 3 minute, increasing the speed.

C. Syrup

Combine the water with the sweetener (honey/brown sugar), mix until its dissolve.

D. Assembly

Put one dough piece add syrup on it and then add 1/3 of the cream. Level the cream and then add another piece of dough that will go to the same process as the first. For the last piece add cream on the side as well.

Put the cake in the fridge for 8hours, or overnight.

3. Nutritional facts (amount per 100g):
Contains Vitamin A, C, calcium, iron
Calories: 147
    Calories from Fat: 53
Total Fat: 5.9g
    Saturated Fat: 3.4g
Cholesterol: 20mg
Sodium: 111mg
Potassium: 92mg
Total Carbohydrates: 28.8g
    Sugar: 2.2g
Protein: 7.2g

36. Apple desert

Preparing time: 10 minutes
Cooking time: 35-40 minutes
Servings: 9

1. Ingredients:

- Dough

80g oats flour
120g black rice flour
15g corn starch
7g baking powder
70g sweetener (honey/brown sugar)
220g apple puree
150ml coconut milk
2 eggs whites
1 teaspoon cinnamon (5g)

- Topping

400g apples
200ml water
50ml milk
50g sweetener (honey/brown sugar)
4 sheets gelatin
½ teaspoon cinnamon (2.5g)

2. Preparation:

A. Dough

Mix the oat flour with the rice flour, starch, baking powder, sweetener (honey/brown sugar) and cinnamon. Add the apple puree, coconut milk, egg whites and mix for 3-4minutes.

Put the composition in a tray and cook it for 35-40minutes in a preheated oven at 180degree Celsius.

B. Topping

Put the gelatin sheet in cold water.

In a frying pan put the slice apple and water, milk, sweetener (honey/brown sugar) and cinnamon and boil for about 15minutes at low heat.

Add the gelatin sheets and mix till there dissolve. Wait till it cool down.

Pour the topping on to the dough and put it in the fridge for 6hours or in the freezer for 1hour.

3. *Nutritional facts (amount per 100g):*
Contains Vitamin C, calcium, iron
Calories: 120
    Calories from Fat: 29
Total Fat: 3.2g
    Saturated Fat: 2.5g
Cholesterol: 0mg
Sodium: 15mg
Potassium: 148mg

Total Carbohydrates: 28.9g
    Sugar: 5.2g
Protein: 4.7g

37. Coconut cookies

Preparing time: 5 minutes
Cooking time: 15-20 minutes

1. Ingredients:

100g coconut flour
50g black rice flour
15g flour (white)
30g whey protein
7g baking powder
70g sweetener (honey/brown sugar)
15ml coconut oil
250ml coconut milk
2 egg whites
1 teaspoon coconut essence (5g)
1 teaspoon butter essence (5g)

2. Preparation:

Mix the coconut flour with the rice flour and the plain flour. Add the whey protein, baking powder and sweetener (honey/brown sugar).

Melt some coconut oil and add it to the composition. Mix well

Add the coconut milk, eggs whites, and essence, and mix till you have a dough.

Roll the dough on a clean surface and then with a glass make round shapes in it.

Place the result in tray (whit a baking sheet in). And add them in the preheated oven at 180degree Celsius for 15-20minutes.

3. *Nutritional facts (amount per 100g):*
Contains Vitamin C, calcium, iron
Calories: 255
    Calories from Fat: 131
Total Fat: 14.6g
    Saturated Fat: 12.3g
Cholesterol: 10mg
Sodium: 27mg
Potassium: 285mg
Total Carbohydrates: 37.6g
    Sugar: 1.7g
Protein: 8.8g

38. Dark chocolate cookies

Preparing time: 5 minutes
Cooking time: 15 minutes
Servings: 20

1. Ingredients:

60g black rice flour
60g oats flour
50g whey protein
50g sweetener (honey/brown sugar)
15g corn starch
10g baking powder
1 teaspoon vanilla
1 egg
1 egg white
50ml coconut milk
½ tablespoon chocolate flavor (7g)
40g dark chocolate

2. Preparation:

Mix the oat flour with the rice flour, whey protein, starch, baking powder, vanilla and sweetener (honey/brown sugar).

Add egg, egg white, coconut milk, chocolate essence and mix till smooth.

Chop the chocolate in small pieces. Add it to the composition.

Whit the help of a teaspoon take dough and place on the baking tray.

Bake the cookies in a preheated oven at 180degree Celsius for 15minutes.

3. *Nutritional facts (amount per 20g):*
Contains calcium, iron;
Calories: 57
   Calories from Fat: 16
Total Fat: 1.8g
   Saturated Fat: 1.2g
Cholesterol: 14mg
Sodium: 12mg
Potassium: 98mg
Total Carbohydrates: 10.1g
   Sugar: 1.2g
Protein: 3.1g

39. Chocolate and coconut flakes cake

Preparing time: 5 minutes
Waiting time: 60 minutes

1. Ingredients:
300g powder milk
14g cocoa powder
200ml milk
30g sweetener (honey/brown sugar)
10g coconut flakes
1 teaspoon coconut essence (5g)

2. Preparation:

In a bowl add the powder milk and cocoa and mix till there combine.

In 200ml milk add sweetener (honey/brown sugar) and coconut essence. The milk needs to be warm.

Add the milk on the powder milk and mix till smoothen.

In a silicon shape put the coconut flakes and then pour the composition over it. Put the form in the freezer for 1hour.

3. Nutritional facts (amount per 100g):
Contains Vitamin A, calcium, iron;
Calories: 280
    Calories from Fat: 141

Total Fat: 15.6g
   Saturated Fat: 1.1g
Cholesterol: 3mg
Sodium: 167mg
Potassium: 679mg
Total Carbohydrates: 29.4g
   Sugar: 1.7g
Protein: 12.5g

40. Chocolate balls

Preparing time: 10 minutes
Cooking time: 30 minutes
Servings: 15

1. Ingredients:
50g cocoa butter
50g sweetener (honey/brown sugar)
50g whey protein (chocolate)
18g cocoa powder
30g powder milk
Pinch of salt

2. Preparation:

Melt the butter. Add sweetener (honey/brown sugar), whey protein, cocoa, milk powder and mix till smooth.

Pour the composition in form whit praline shapes.

Put the form in the freezer for 30minutes.

3. Nutritional facts (amount per 10g):
Contains Vitam A, calcium, iron
Calories: 61
    Calories from Fat: 43
Total Fat: 4.7g
Cholesterol: 7mg
Sodium: 24mg
Potassium: 73mg

Total Carbohydrates: 5.8g
Protein: 3g

41. Mango cheesecake

Preparing time: 1 hour
Waiting time: 4-5 hours
Servings: 10

1. Ingredients:

200g mango (2 fruits)
3 tablespoon lemon juice
800g cottage cheese
200g sour cream
100g powdered sugar
1 teaspoon vanilla essence (15g)
150g butter
200g digestive biscuits
15g gelatin
100g mix nuts

2. Preparation:

The mangos are blended together with the lemon juice. The composition (manga puree) is passed through a strainer.

Melt the butter and add the mesh biscuits, mix till you have a dough and add it to a tray.

In two small bowls dived the gelatin (10g in the first 5g in the second). Add water in each.

The sour cream is mix till it becomes whipped cream.

The cottage cheese is mix for 1-2 minutes, till it's becomes a cream.

Split the mango puree in two bowls in one of them add 10g gelatin and mix till its dissolve.

3 tablespoon of cottage cheese cream is added on the mango and gelatin bowl. Mix well. Then add the cheese cream, whipped cream and sugar, there mix until smooth.

Pour the composition on to the dough and put it into the freeze.

After the cheese cream has hardened (after 15-20 minutes in the freezer) mix the rest of the mango puree with the remaining gelatin and add it on the surface. Add the cake to the fridge for 2hours.

For decoration use the mix nuts, mint leaf, caramel syrup or chocolate syrup.

3. Nutritional facts (amount per 100g):
Contains Vitamin A, C, calcium, iron
Calories: 245
    Calories from Fat: 143
Total Fat: 15.9g
    Saturated Fat: 7.2g
Cholesterol: 29mg
Sodium: 312mg

Potassium: 90mg
Total Carbohydrates: 17.3g
    Sugar: 10.4g
Protein: 9g

42. Brownie

Preparing time: 10 minutes
Cooking time: 1 hour
Servings: 10

1. Ingredients:

- Dough

210g flour

60g cocoa powder

250g butter

3 eggs

330ml black beer

125g white sugar

200g brown sugar

Pinch of salt

2 teaspoons vanilla essence (10g)

1 teaspoon cinnamon (5g)

100g dark chocolate

20g almonds

50g raisins

- Topping

300ml sour cream

50g brown sugar

1 teaspoon vanilla essence

2. Preparation:

Heat the oven at 180degree Celsius. The tray that you will use greases with hard butter and sprinkle it with flower.

In a bowl add flour, cocoa, baking powder, cinnamon and salt. Mix till there combine.

Mix the butter for 1 minute. Add sugar, and mix for 3 minutes. Add eggs and vanilla extract and mix for another minute.

Add the flour composition and the black beer gradually. Add the nuts and chocolate.

Put the composition in the grease tray.

Put it in the oven for 45-55 minutes.

3. Nutritional facts (amount per 100g):
Contains Vitamin A, calcium, iron;
Calories: 322
    Calories from Fat: 158
Total Fat: 17.6g
    Saturated Fat: 10.6g
Cholesterol: 64mg
Sodium: 115mg
Potassium: 203mg
Total Carbohydrates: 38.5g
    Sugar: 25.4g
Protein: 4.1g

43. Fruit bars

Preparing time: 20 minutes
Waiting time: 1 hour
Servings: 24

1. Ingredients:

200g oats
50g corn flakes
4 tablespoons honey (60g)
50g whey protein
150g brown sugar
60g white chocolate
100g butter
80g cranberries
10g raisins
20g raspberry
20g currants

2. Preparation:

Melt the butter with brown sugar, whey protein and honey. Add the white chocolate, mixing till its dissolve.

Once the chocolate its dissolve add the flakes and the fruits. Mix well.

In a tray add a baking sheet and then put the composition in and level it. Put it in the fridge for an hour.

After they cool down cut the bars.

3. Nutritional facts (amount per 35g):
Contains Vitamin A, C, calcium, iron
Calories: 129
   Calories from Fat: 44
Total Fat: 4.8g
   Saturated Fat: 2.8g
Cholesterol: 14mg
Sodium: 52mg
Potassium: 75mg
Total Carbohydrates: 19g
   Sugar: 11.2g
Protein: 3g

44. Cheese and marshmallow tart

Preparing time: 1 hour
Waiting time: 3 hours

1. Ingredients:

250g digestive biscuit

50g butter

4 yolks

170g brown sugar

20g vanilla sugar

50g starch

450ml milk (warm)

1 tablespoon gelatin (15g)

250g cottage cheese

300g dried apricots

4 eggs whites

100g sugar

2. Preparation:

A. Dough

Melt the butter and mesh the biscuits. Then combine the two and mix until you have a "dough". Mold the dough in a round tray. Put it in the fridge for 30minutes.

B. Cream

Put the gelatin in water.

Mix the yolks with sugar and vanilla sugar. Then add starch mixing continue until smoothen.

Add the warm milk on the composition. Then put the composition on the oven at low heat, mixing continue, till it's thickens. Remove from the oven.

Add the cottage cheese and mix till you have a soft cream.

Add the gelatin and mix till its dissolve.

C. Assembly

On the dough place the apricots. Then place the cream on top and put it in the fridge immediately.

The egg whites are mix in a soft foam then the sugar is added and mix till the foam hardens. The foam is place with a tablespoon on the cake.

The cake goes into the fridge for 3hours.

3. Nutritional facts (amount per 100g):
Contains Vitamin A, C, calcium, iron
Calories: 208
    Calories from Fat: 67
Total Fat: 7.4g
    Saturated Fat: 2.9g
Cholesterol: 59mg
Sodium: 166mg
Potassium: 111mg
Total Carbohydrates: 30.5g

Sugar: 22.1g
Protein: 5.9g

45. Banana biscuit

Preparing time: 15 minutes
Cooking time: 10 minutes
Servings: 60-70

1. Ingredients:

2 bananas
2 tablespoon lemon juice (30g)
50g egg white (from 2-3 eggs)
200g brown sugar
70g whey protein
1 teaspoon vanilla essence (5g)
10g baking powder
200g oats flour
Pinch of salt
120ml oil
100g dehydrated banana

2. Preparation:

Mash the bananas, and then add the juice from the lemon and mix. Then put the egg whites, whey protein and brown sugar.

Mix at a medium speed for 3-4 minutes and you will obtain foam. Then add the vanilla essence and oil mixing continue.

Last add the flour and the baking powder and mix till smooth.

Preheat the oven at 180degree Celsius.

Whit a teaspoon form discs of 5cm wide on the tray. On every disc put dehydrated bananas.

Cook for 8-10 minutes.

3. *Nutritional facts (amount per 15g):*
Contains Vitamin A, C, calcium, iron
Calories: 49
    Calories from Fat: 17
Total Fat: 1.9g
Cholesterol: 2mg
Sodium: 7mg
Potassium: 69mg
Total Carbohydrates: 7.1g
    Sugar: 3.9g
Protein: 1.3g

46. Forest fruit pancakes

Preparing time: 10 minutes
Cooking time: 15 minutes
Servings: 3

1. Ingredients:

250g oat flour

2 tablespoon brown sugar (30g)

200ml milk

2 tablespoons butter (30g)

5g baking powder

2 eggs

Pinch of salt

1 teaspoons vanilla essence (5g)

150g fruits (raspberry, blackberries, currants)

Honey and maple syrup for topping

2. Preparation:

In a bowl add flour, sugar, and baking powder.

Mix the egg whites with the salt till they form hard foam.

And the yolks are mixt with milk and then added in the flour bowl with the vanilla essence, butter (melted) and the egg whites.

Mix the composition well, the result needs to be semi-hard dough (not foamy).

Sugar: 1.4g
Protein: 26.1g

48. Strawberry marshmallow cream

Preparing time: 40 minutes
Cooking time: 10 minutes

1. Ingredients:

400g strawberries
350g brown sugar
150g egg whites (5 eggs)
70g whey protein
Pinch of salt
375g butter (at room temperature)
20ml lemon juice
1 tablespoon vanilla essence (15g)

2. Preparation:

Slice the strawberries and put them in a frying pan, put them on the oven at medium heat. Leave them there till they soften then add 300g brown sugar and mix them with a blender. Lower the heat and leave them on the oven.

Mix the eggs whites with the salt, until they form a soft foam, then add the reaming sugar and whey protein and mix again until the foam hardens.

Put the strawberries in the foam and mix continue. Mix till the composition begins to cools down.

After it reach the room temperature the butter is added, piece by piece and mixing continue. AT the end add the vanilla essence. And mix for a few more seconds.

If you feel that the creams cuts put the bowl in the fridge for about 15-20minuts after mix at a high speed.

3. *Nutritional facts (amount per 100g):*
Contains Vitamin A, C, iron, calcium;
Calories: 349
    Calories from Fat: 215
Total Fat: 23.8g
    Saturated Fat: 15g
Cholesterol: 73mg
Sodium: 207mg
Potassium: 142mg
Total Carbohydrates: 29.7g
    Sugar: 28.1g
Protein: 5.6g

49. Strawberry pancakes

Preparing time: 5 minutes
Cooking time: 10 minutes
Servings: 8

1. Ingredients:

2 bananas

100g almond flour

50g flour

40g whey protein

3 eggs

½ teaspoon vanilla essence (2.5g)

½ cup mineral water (120ml)

100g strawberries

2. Preparation:

Mix the banana in a blender. Add the rest of the ingredients and mix till the composition becomes creamy.

In a pan add some butter and start adding composition.

Blend the strawberries and add them as a topping on the pancakes.

3. Nutritional facts (amount per 100g):
Contains Vitamin A, C, iron, calcium;
Calories: 117
    Calories from Fat: 35
Total Fat: 3.9g

    Saturated Fat: 0.8g
Cholesterol: 72mg
Sodium: 40mg
Potassium: 182mg
Total Carbohydrates: 14g
    Sugar: 4.7g
Protein: 7.5g

50. Cheesecake with chocolate, cocoas and avocado

Preparing time: 20 minutes
Waiting time: 6 hours

1. Ingredients:
- Dough

200g persimmon

100g coconut

- Cream

500g mascarpone

Juice from 1 lime (20ml)

200g dark chocolate

2 tablespoon cocoa powder (30g)

100ml coconut milk

2 avocados

- Jelly

1 cup raspberries (120g)

200ml milk

20g gelatin

- Decor

Strawberries

White chocolate flakes

2. Preparation:
A. Dough

Let the persimmon hydrated overnight in water.

Mix the coconut till you obtain coconut flacks. Then add the persimmon and mix till the texture become creamy. The paste will be place on a tray and put in the fridge.

B. Cream

Melt the chocolate in the microwave or at bain-marie.

Mix the mascarpone cream with the coconut milk and lime juice. Add the two avocados (mixed beforehand) and mix till smooth. Add the chocolate and the cocoa powder.

The composition is place on the dough and put it in the fridge.

C. Jelly

Mix the fruits with a blander add the milk and the gelatin and mix till its smooth.

Pour it over the composition from the fridge.

For the décor use the chocolate flakes and strawberries.

3. Nutritional facts (amount per 100g):
Contains Vitamin A, C, iron, calcium;
Calories: 215
    Calories from Fat: 134
Total Fat: 14.8g
    Saturated Fat: 8.6g
Cholesterol: 18mg
Sodium: 43mg

Potassium: 281mg
Total Carbohydrates: 16.1g
    Sugar: 7.3g
Protein: 6.3g

51. Chocolate and avocado pudding

Preparing time: 5 minutes
Servings: 2

1. Ingredients:

1 avocado

400g coconut milk

50g coconut flour

70g cocoa powder

60g sweetener (honey/brown sugar)

1 teaspoon vanilla essence (5g)

10g forest fruits

2. Preparation:

All the ingredients beside the fruits are put in a blender and mix for 5minutus. The result should be a dense cream.

Put them in recipients and add the forest fruit on top.

3. Nutritional facts (amount per 100g):

Contains Vitamin A, C, iron, calcium;
Calories: 216
    Calories from Fat: 168
Total Fat: 18.6g
    Saturated Fat: 12.7g
Cholesterol: 0mg
Sodium: 11mg
Potassium: 474mg

Total Carbohydrates: 23.5g
  Sugar: 2.5g
Protein: 4.1g

52. Oat brownie

Preparing time: 10 minutes
Cooking time: 40-45 minutes
Servings:

1. Ingredients:

100g raisins

20g cocoa powder

4 eggs

15g starch

250g Greek yogurt

70g sweetener (honey/brown sugar)

100g oats

50g almonds

1 teaspoons vanilla essence (5g)

2. Preparation:

In a bowl mix cocoa powder, raisins and eggs. Add yogurt, sweetener (honey/brown sugar), starch, baking powder and vanilla.

The oats and almond are grinded and the added to the composition.

Put them in a tray and cook them for 40-45minutes at 180degrees Celsius.

3. Nutritional facts (amount per 100g):

Contains Vitamin A, calcium, iron;
Calories: 189
    Calories from Fat: 64
Total Fat: 7.2g
    Saturated Fat: 1.7g
Cholesterol: 83mg
Sodium: 44mg
Potassium: 322mg
Total Carbohydrates: 34.5g
    Sugar: 9.3g
Protein: 9.7g

53. Yogurt cake

Preparing time: 2-3 hours

1. Ingredients:
200g digestive biscuits
½ cup sugar (120g)
200g Greek yogurt
100g milk
1 teaspoon vanilla essence (5g)
10g gelatin
100g prunes

2. Preparation:

Mix the yogurt with the sugar, vanilla and the prunes (slice in small bites). Add the gelatin (melted in hot water).

On a tray place a food foil and on it place the digestive biscuits (dipped in milk) then add a layer of yogurt composition then again biscuits, and last a layer of yogurt. Cover it with the food foil and put it in the fridge.

Leave it in the fridge till the composition hardens.

3. Nutritional facts (amount per 100g):
Contains Vitamin A, calcium, iron;
Calories: 258
    Calories from Fat: 68
Total Fat: 7.6g

Saturated Fat: 2g
Cholesterol: 10mg
Sodium: 159mg
Potassium: 175mg
Total Carbohydrates: 42.4g
    Sugar: 28.6g
Protein: 6.5g

54. Banana desert

Preparing time: 10 minutes
Baking time: 30 minutes

1. Ingredients:
½ cup flour (120g)
½ cup sugar (120g)
½ cup milk (120g)
30g whey protein
1 tablespoon butter (15g)
2g baking powder
3 bananas
2 eggs

2. Preparation:

Mix the butter with the sugar then add the eggs, whey protein, bananas and milk. Mix till the dough is smooth and add the flour and the baking powder.

Put the mix in a tray and put it in the oven at 180degree Celsius for about 30minutes.

3. Nutritional facts (amount per 100g):
Contains Vitamin A, C, calcium, iron;
Calories: 166
    Calories from Fat: 30
Total Fat: 3.3g

Saturated Fat: 1.6g
Cholesterol: 54mg
Sodium: 40mg
Potassium: 237mg
Total Carbohydrates: 30g
　　Sugar: 18.8g
Protein: 5.9g

55. Yolk cupcakes

Preparing time: 1 day
Servings: 6

1. Ingredients:

5 eggs
1 tablespoon butter (15g)
1 tablespoon vanilla essence
100g chocolate flakes
100g sugar
100g raisins

2. Preparation:

Boil the eggs. They should be hard so you should let them boil for about 10 minutes.

Remove the yolks and mesh them with a fork. Add the butter, vanilla, chocolate flakes, and sugar.

Mix till smoothen and add the composition in cupcakes shapes put the raisins on top of them.

Put them in the fridge and leave them overnight.

3. Nutritional facts (amount per 100g):

Contains Vitamin A, C, calcium, iron
Calories: 296
    Calories from Fat: 70
Total Fat: 7.8g
    Saturated Fat: 3.3g

Cholesterol: 170mg
Sodium: 165mg
Potassium: 213mg
Total Carbohydrates: 49.5g
    Sugar: 36.5g
Protein: 8.2g

56. Cookie cheesecake

Preparing time: 4 hours
Baking time: 10-15 minutes

1. Ingredients:

200g digestive biscuits
100g butter
1 teaspoon vanilla essence (15g)
400g cottage cheese
1 lemon
100g brown sugar
4 eggs
200g currants

2. Preparation:

For the dough: mash the biscuits in the melted butter, mix. Put the composition in a tray and distribute it equal on the surface. Put the tray in the fridge for a couple of hours 3-4.

For the cream: Mix the cheese with the rind and juice from the lemon, sugar, vanilla and the egg yolks. In another bowl you mill mix the egg whites, when they are forming foam you can put them over the yolks.

Remove the dough from the fridge and add the cream over it and cook it for 10-15minutes at 180 degree Celsius (the cream has to change color).

Removed from the oven and add the currants on top.

3. *Nutritional facts (amount per 100g):*
Contains Vitamin A, C, calcium, iron
Calories: 233
    Calories from Fat: 115
Total Fat: 12.8g
    Saturated Fat: 5.9g
Cholesterol: 79mg
Sodium: 288mg
Potassium: 130mg
Total Carbohydrates: 22.2g
    Sugar: 13.8g
Protein: 7.8g

57. Banana shuffle

Preparing time: 10 minutes
Baking time: 30 minutes

1. Ingredients:

3 bananas
50g whey protein
½ lemon (the lemon juice from ½ lemon)
3 eggs whites
Sweetener (honey/brown sugar) per taste
1 teaspoon vanilla essence (5g)

2. Preparation:

Mash the bananas and add the lemon juice and the vanilla essence in a bowl.

In a separate bowl add the egg whites are mix until there become foam and then you add the sweetener (honey/brown sugar) and whey protein slowly.

Combine the 2 compositions and mix until they smooth.

Add them in shapes and cook them in the preheated oven at 180degrees Celsius for 30minutes.

3. Nutritional facts (amount per 100g):
Contains Vitamin A, C, calcium, iron
Calories: 114

Calories from Fat: 8
Total Fat: 0.9g
Cholesterol: 21mg
Sodium: 39mg
Potassium: 344mg
Total Carbohydrates: 27g
    Sugar: 9.2g
Protein: 10.1g

58. Nuts cookies

Preparing time: 5 minutes
Baking time: 15 minutes
Servings: 12

1. Ingredients:

85g nuts

1 egg

50g whey protein

1 tablespoon vanilla essence

1 tablespoon almond essence

20-30g sweetener (honey/brown sugar)

2. Preparation:

Grind the nuts and mix them with the eggs, whey protein, essence and sweetener (honey/brown sugar). Add the composition in muffin forms and put them in the preheated oven at 180degrees Celsius for 15minutes.

3. Nutritional facts (amount per 20g):
Contains Vitamin A, C, calcium, iron
Calories: 69
    Calories from Fat: 38
Total Fat: 4.2g
    Saturated Fat: 0.7g
Cholesterol: 22mg
Sodium: 60mg
Potassium: 73mg

Total Carbohydrates: 5.4g
 Sugar: 0.6g
Protein: 4.7g

59. Cottage cheese donuts

Preparing time: 1:45 hours
Baking time: 20 minutes
Servings: 9-10

1. Ingredients:

250g flour
225g cottage cheese
100g milk (warm)
40g brown sugar
15g yeast
1 tablespoon vanilla sugar (15g)
Rind from a lemon and an orange

2. Preparation:

Mix the flour with the yeast and add the cottage cheese in, the warm milk, sugar, vanilla sugar and rind. Mix till the composition is homogeny.

Leave the dough in a plastic bowl covered with aluminum foil, in a warm place, for about 45minutes.

After 45 minutes roll the dough with your hands in a sheet about 1-1,5 cm thick.

Whit the help of a glass make donuts shapes, and place them on a tray.

Leave them in the tray for another 45minutes and they put them in the preheated oven at 200 degree Celsius for 20minutes.

After they cool down powder them with vanilla sugar.

3. Nutritional facts (amount per 50g):
Contains calcium, iron
Calories: 117
    Calories from Fat: 7
Total Fat: 0.8g
Cholesterol: 2mg
Sodium: 82mg
Potassium: 75mg
Total Carbohydrates: 21.7g
    Sugar: 4.7g
Protein: 5.5g

60. Pears and nuts desert

Preparing time: 15 minutes
Baking time: 40 minutes

1. Ingredients:

280g flour

75g coconut flakes

150g brown sugar

100ml sunflower oil

250ml warm milk

300g pears

60g mix of nuts

1 tablespoons baking powder (15g)

1-2 teaspoons cinnamon (5-10g)

Pinch of salt

2. Preparation:

In a bowl mix the sugar with oil and milk, add flour and baking powder, salt and last the coconut flakes.

Mix till the composition is smooth and then the nuts (mesh), cinnamon and pears (slice in squares).

Grease a round tray (or a square one) with butter and add a coat of flour on it and add the dough.

Preheat the oven at 180degree Celsius and leave it to cook for about 40-45minutes.

3. Nutritional facts (amount per 100g):

Contains Vitamin A, C, iron, calcium
Calories: 283
    Calories from Fat: 123
Total Fat: 13.6g
    Saturated Fat: 3.3g
Cholesterol: 2mg
Sodium: 47mg
Potassium: 232mg
Total Carbohydrates: 37.5g
    Sugar: 16.2g
Protein: 4.3g

OTHER GREAT TITLES BY THIS AUTHOR

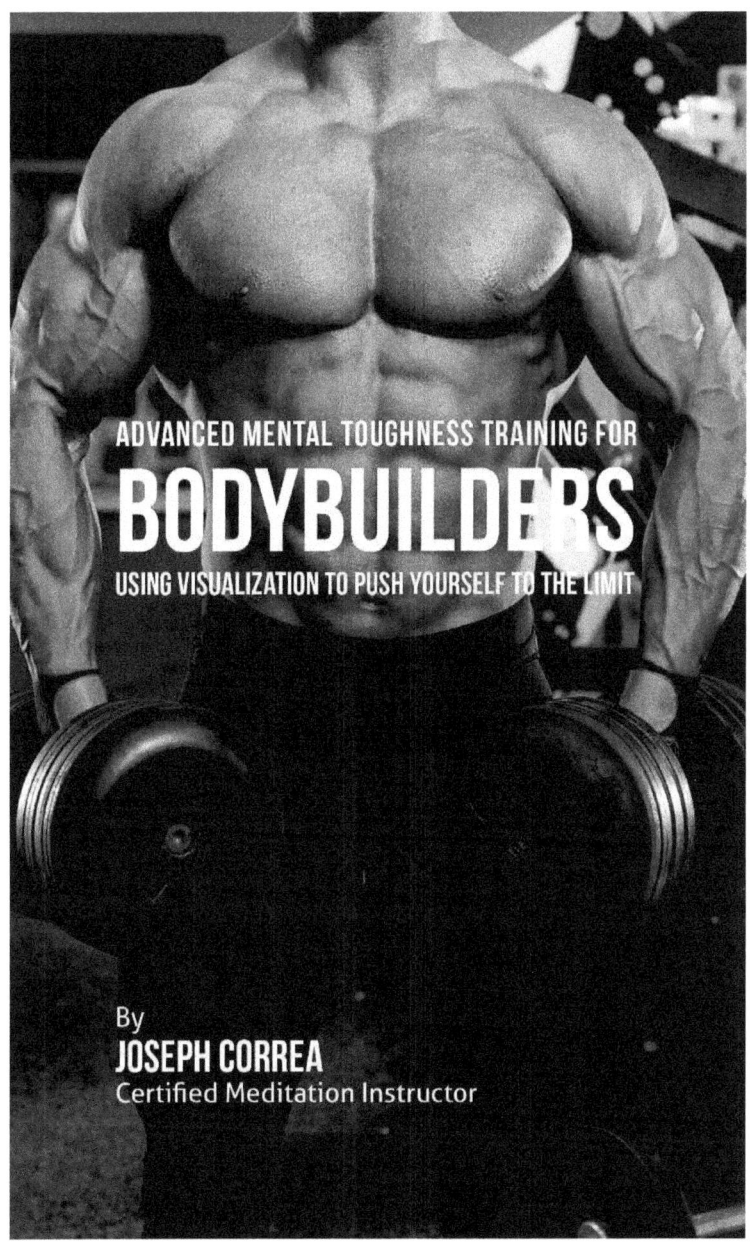

www.ingramcontent.com/pod-product-compliance
Lightning Source LLC
Chambersburg PA
CBHW071715020426
42333CB00017B/2285